KETOGENIC DIET PLAN

Please note the information contained within this document is for educational and entertainment purposes only. All effort has been executed to present accurate, up to date, reliable, complete information. No warranties of any kind are declared or implied. Readers acknowledge that the author is not engaged in the rendering of legal, financial, medical, or professional advice. The content within this book has been derived from various sources. Please consult a licensed professional before attempting any techniques outlined in this book.

By reading this document, the reader agrees that under no circumstances is the author responsible for any losses, direct or indirect, that are incurred because of the use of the information contained within this document, including, but not limited to, errors, omissions, or inaccuracies.

Table of Contents

Introduction

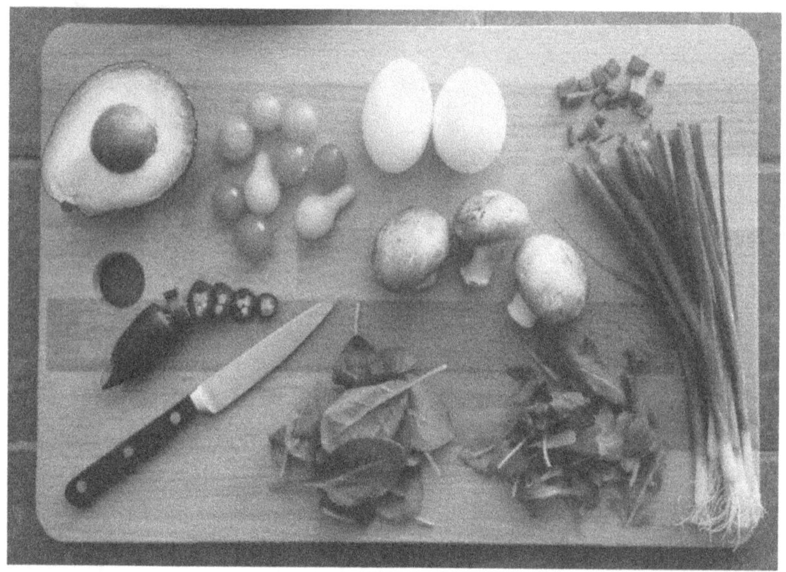

Are you looking to make a fresh start in your eating habits? Are you overweight or struggling with any health issues? Perhaps your doctor has told you that you need to change your diet or that you are eating your way to illness?

Diets can be so stressful and finding the one that best suits your lifestyle, and your taste buds can be extremely challenging. If you are the type of person who gets demotivated by slow progress, then the keto lifestyle might be just what you are looking for as this diet allows for rapid weight loss in a short period of time. Seeing yourself shed a few pounds each week will help you stay motivated. Exercise is encouraged, but you do not need to do extraneous exercises to get results. Essentially, the ketogenic diet offers variety in taste and has effective short and long-term health benefits.

The ketogenic diet is a high fat, adequate protein, and low carb diet that works similar to fasting by getting your body into a metabolic condition called ketosis. If you have tried diet regimes like intermittent fasting, you will know the benefits of ketosis in helping with weight loss. Because intermittent fasting can be difficult to stick to, the ketogenic diet offers a solution. When you are on a keto diet, not only are there no restrictions on when you eat, but the food you do eat will allow you to stay in ketosis longer aiding in weight loss. If you have heard about the benefits of intermittent fasting and ketogenesis, this is the diet you should acquaint yourself with.

Not only is the ketogenic diet great for weight loss, but it also has some significant health benefits as dieticians now link this diet to improvements in treating diabetes. There are also the other benefits of eating healthier in general and as such this diet will have you feeling amazing throughout the day as it increases your overall energy level.

The ketogenic diet is one diet that lives up to its promises and when you look at how it works, it makes sense why it works. Of course, you need to find a diet that works best for you, but the ketogenic diet is easily doable once you understand it. This book reveals some of the science behind the ketogenic diet to help with this understanding. This book also provides recipes to help you prepare a variety of meals that not only will your taste buds dance to but will also help you stay on this diet for longer than expected. Diets are never easy, but if you commit yourself to the keto diet you will see noticeable changes in your mood, energy, and body composition within weeks.

To combat both ageing and the junk food we are constantly surrounded by, we need to work together with our bodies to ensure they perform optimally. There are many diseases that are now being shown to have a direct link to our diets. This does not mean we need to eat like rabbits munching on greens all day, we can still have the occasional treat, but we do need to think about what we are putting in our bodies. The ketogenic diet allows you to lower the intake of harmful foods, increase the intake of helpful foods, and it does so without neglecting the taste buds.

Chapter 1: What is the Ketogenic Diet?

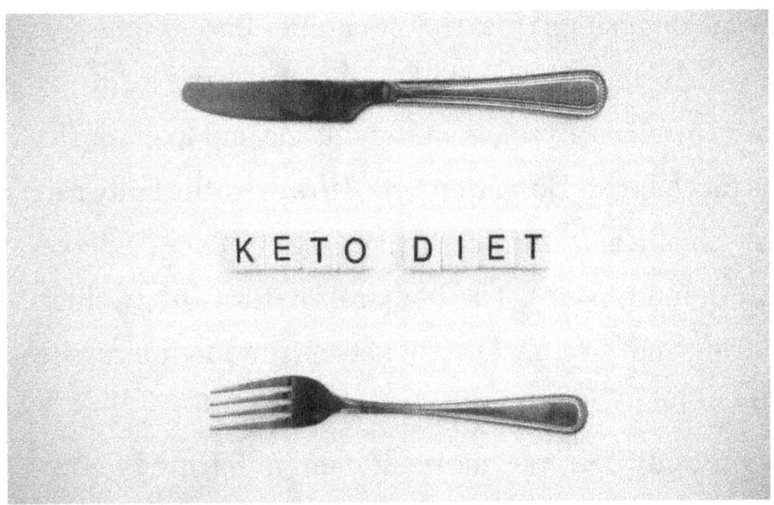

The ketogenic diet, also known as the keto diet, is a low-carb, high fat, and adequate protein diet. While you are on it, you are expected to drastically reduce your carbohydrate intake to close to zero and replace it with fat. This reduction in carbohydrates and increase in fat intake gears your body to experience a metabolic action called ketosis. Therefore, the ketogenic diet is metabolically like fasting. It attempts to mimic the effects of fasting (which is getting the body into ketosis), however, it does this by allowing you to still consume food regularly.

What is Ketosis?

The body has three storage deposits of fuel that it can tap into for energy. It can use (1) proteins, which can be converted to glucose in the liver, (2) carbohydrates, which are stored as glycogen in the muscle and liver, or (3) fats, which are stored as fat cells (McDonald, 1998). However, the body can also survive on ketones—chemicals your liver makes that replaces glucose as a fat-derived fuel (McDonald, 1998). The body rarely turns to produce ketones for energy under normal circumstances; ketone production can be invoked by either fasting or being on the ketogenic diet.

When ketosis occurs, your body becomes more efficient at burning fat for fuel by turning it into ketones in the liver. In fact, the average person has enough energy stored as body fat to survive for two weeks without eating (McDonald, 1998). Under ketosis, your body is in a high fat burning state and, as a result, you lose weight. This sole aspect of the ketogenic diet is what attracts many fitness fanatics to the diet because they are assured to lose body fat instead of muscle mass.

The primary role of ketones in the body is to replace glucose as fuel for the brain should a person go into fasting or a starved state. Previously, some scientists believed that the brain could only properly function on glucose. However, it has been found that the brain can easily function on ketones when a person has not had food to eat in a while, or when a person is fasting. This implies that it is safe for our body to depend upon ketones for day-to-day functioning and survival. Another key role of ketones is to prevent protein breakdown of the body when a person is starving. Ketogenesis kicks in to prevent protein breakdown, which can be detrimental. Therefore, ketosis is a state that the body naturally shifts to when circumstances allow it—it is a 100% natural process that need not be feared.

Ketosis is sparked by a decrease in insulin and an increase in glycogen. When insulin levels are high, which normally happens when you eat a high carb meal, fat storage kicks in due to the disproportionate number of calories you are consuming compared to what you are burning off through physical activity. By ingesting sugary drinks and a high-carb diet, one is likely to gain weight because insulin levels will always be spiked.

Ketogenesis happens in fat cells and the liver. The liver is always producing ketones in small amounts, which can be found in the bloodstream. When on the ketogenic diet and in a state of ketosis, more ketones can be found in the bloodstream. Some people will even notice a change in the smell of their breath and urine—it will start to smell fruity because of the acetone leaving the body. This is an easy tell to know if your body has entered ketosis.

What Should You Be Eating?

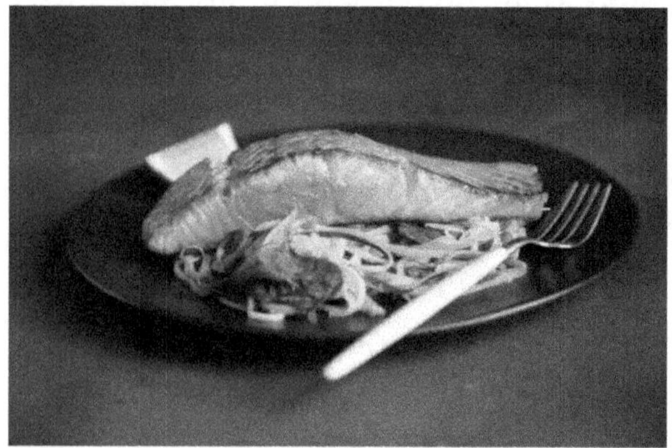

Eating fish and shellfish is highly recommended on the keto diet. Although shellfish like shrimp and crab do not have carbs there are other shellfish which do. These carb shellfish are not forbidden on the diet as they contain little carbs; however, it is important to understand how much they contain so that you do not end up going over the minimal carbohydrate intake for the day and risk getting out of ketosis.

The following is a list of shellfish that are known to contain carbs:

- clams: 4 grams
- octopus: 4 grams
- mussels: 4 grams
- squid: 3 grams
- oysters: 3 grams

(Spritzler, 2020)

Spritzler (2020) also recommends that you consider including salmon, sardines, mackerel, and other fatty fishes, which contain omega 3 fatty acids, as they have been found to lower insulin levels and promote insulin sensitivity in overweight and obese people.

Vegetables

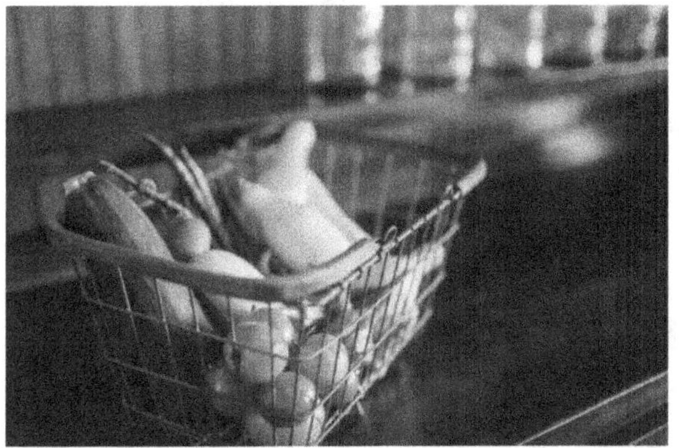

It may not be obvious that some vegetables, like potatoes, contain high levels of carbohydrates. As such, it would do best to stay away from vegetables like potatoes because eating even one boiled potato can spike your carbohydrate intake in each day. It is best to stay away from all starchy vegetables. Non-starchy vegetables are not only a better option because they are low in carbs, but they pack higher nutrient and mineral levels, as well (Spritzler, 2020).

Starting a keto diet will naturally increase your vegetable intake—a food group rich in antioxidants which get rid of free radicals that can cause cell damage. Spritzler (2020) notes vegetables like broccoli, kale, and cauliflower have been linked to decreased cancer and heart disease. Vegetables, however, do contain a lot of fibre which is not easily digested and absorbed in the stomach. Keeping an eye on the labels that state "net carbs" allows you to see the total carbs that your body can absorb.

Vegetables are also great when substituting starchy foods like rice and spaghetti. Yes, it will be a new taste to get used to at first, but with consistency, you should start enjoying the taste of the vegetables and perhaps will never switch back to the original starchy version. Starches like spaghetti can be replaced with spaghetti squash and regular noodles can be replaced with "zoodles" (made from zucchini). If you enjoy rice and mashed potatoes, you could consider using cauliflower. These substitutes will not taste the same, but they help when missing beloved starchy ingredients.

Go-to vegetable list:

- asparagus
- broccoli
- avocado
- cauliflower
- cabbage
- green beans
- cucumber
- kale
- eggplant

- olives

- lettuce

- spinach

- peppers (especially green)

- zucchini

- tomatoes

Cheese

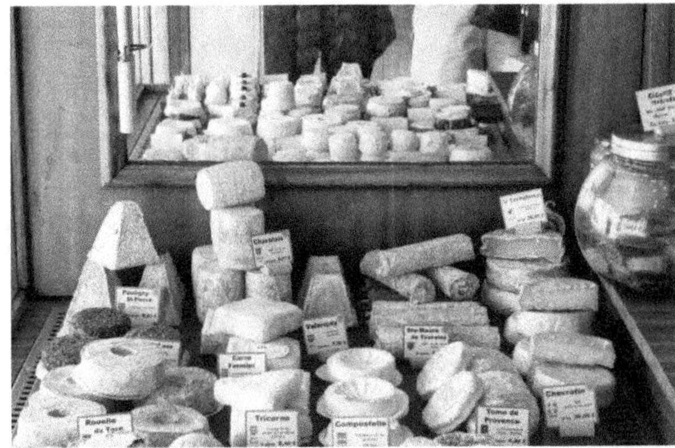

Many kinds of cheese are high in fat and low in carbs, and this makes them a great fit for the ketogenic diet. So, if you are a cheese lover, dig in. Below is a list of cheeses that are low in carbs:

- blue cheese • feta • mozzarella

- camembert • cream cheese   • pepper jack

- brie   • halloumi • parmesan

- chevre
- goat cheese
- romano
- cheddar
- havarti
- provolone
- cottage cheese
- mascarpone

Other Foods Permitted

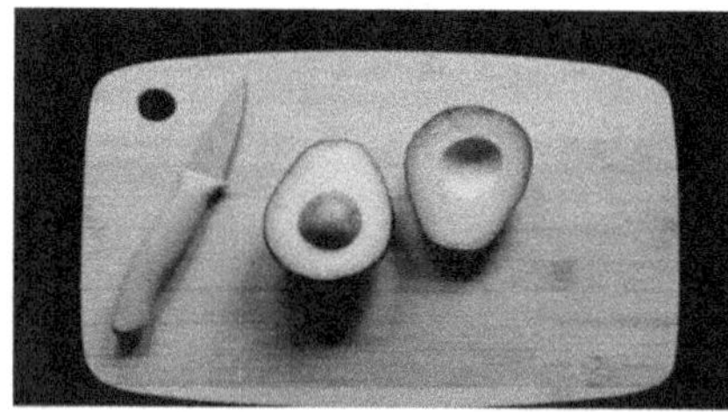 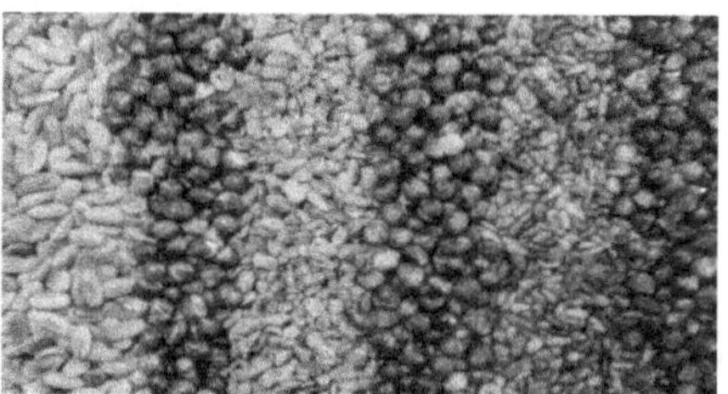

- avocados
- meat and poultry
- eggs
- coconut oil
- plain greek yogurt
- olive oil
- nuts and seeds
- berries
- butter and cream
- olives
- unsweetened coffee and tea
- dark chocolate and cocoa powder

Benefits of the Ketogenic Diet

According to Gunnars (2018), the health benefits of low-carb diets are somewhat controversial. Some people are skeptical of the impact a lowcarb diet has on one's health, considering they are generally high in fat. However, Gunnars notes that there is research to prove that low-carb diets, like the ketogenic diet, have beneficial impacts on one's health both short and long term. The following describes some of the key benefits in his article:

Reduction of Appetite

The reason why most people fall off diets is simple: they get hungry. When your body is used to a high calorie diet and you deprive it of what it is used to, you start feeling hungry. A few days down the line and you feel like you are putting your body through unnecessary strain. This makes you want to quit and head down the street to eat at your favorite fast food joint. Gunnars (2018), argues that the ketogenic diet can help with this hunger sensation as when people eat fewer carbs, and replace that with eating more protein and fat, they are likely to experience less hunger. With hunger out of the way, all that is left to do is stay disciplined and committed to the diet.

Loss of Weight Quickly Right from the Start

Cutting carbs from your diet is by far the most effective way to lose weight. Studies have shown that people who embark on the ketogenic diet lose substantial amounts of weight in a shorter time frame; the first two weeks of the diet will surely have you shedding several pounds. This is due to the diet's effect of reducing water in your body and lowering your insulin levels (the hormone which acts to help your body store fats).

Weight accumulates in different parts of the body and each part can have a different effect on our health. Fat in the abdomen, for instance, indicates that you have fat surrounding your organs. This is dangerous and has been found to lead to complications like heart attacks. Especially in the beginning of the keto diet, individuals will lose most of the initial weight from their abdominal cavity region.

The great thing about the ketogenic diet is that you will lose more weight compared to if you were on other diets, but this weight will be lost without the feeling of hunger. Your appetite will be suppressed as your body switches from using glucose to using ketones for energy. This substantial weight loss can last up to six months, after that, the diet acts like any other diet (Gunnars, 2018). This is because initially the body will go into shock and will slowly adjust to the new eating lifestyle; however, once the body has lost the weight, it will try to retain the current weight. Therefore, you will still lose weight but at a slower rate.

With this information in mind, you may want to take advantage of the initial period of six months. If you can, go hard into the diet—especially if you have a lot of weight to shed. If you do this (and even add a little physical activity), you are likely to reach your goal weight faster.

Decreased Triglycerides Circulating in the Blood

Triglycerides are fat molecules that can be found in the bloodstream. When a person has more of these triglycerides circulating, they are in danger of getting clogged arteries and developing heart problems. The ketogenic diet is a proven way of decreasing triglyceride levels, and when people who live a generally inactive lifestyle follow the ketogenic diet, triglyceride levels are reduced drastically. Although it was formerly believed that the ketogenic diet may have a negative impact on the heart because of its highfat content, when it is compared to other diets, those which are low in fat result in higher levels of triglycerides in the bloodstream.

Increased Levels of Good Cholesterol

The ketogenic diet increases levels of high-density lipoprotein (HDL), which is also known as "good cholesterol". We want higher levels of HDL in our body because this helps to lower the risk of developing heart problems. As such, the best way to improve the levels of this type of cholesterol in your blood is to eat more good fat (such as fat from coconut oil, avocados, olives, etc.). Eating more good fats aids the body by increasing HDL, and low-carb diets like the ketogenic diet are high in this good type of fat.

Improved Bad Cholesterol Levels & Lowered Blood Pressure

People with high levels of bad cholesterol (lower-density lipoprotein or LDL) run the risk of getting heart complications like clogged arteries and heart attacks. A low-carb diet can, therefore, boost your heart health by lowering the amount of LDL in your bloodstream. High blood pressure is also a common disease and when one's blood pressure is too high, it puts a strain on organs like the heart and the liver and can lead to the occurrence of strokes. The old saying, "an apple a day keeps the doctor away", holds true—when you eat healthier, you reduce the risk of many life-threatening illnesses.

Reduced Blood Sugar and Insulin Levels

The ketogenic diet is particularly beneficial for people with diabetes. Diabetes causes high insulin levels which can be drastically reduced with the ketogenic diet. Since carbohydrates and sugar are known for spiking one's insulin levels, if carbohydrate intake is reduced, this will naturally work with one's diabetes medication to regulate blood glucose levels. People with diabetes have given this diet great reviews. Many individuals reduced their glucose levels up to 50% and within six months of initiating the diet, many patients were taken off their medication (Olsen, 2019). However, one should be careful when using a diet as the only means of regulating blood glucose levels. Always consult with a doctor before making any life altering decisions.

Paying attention to our diet will keep us healthy and reduce our chances of losing our lives to lifestyle diseases like diabetes, high blood pressure, and strokes. Diets are not easy, and a low carb diet may not be enticing, but paying close attention to the things we eat goes beyond just wanting to lose weight and look good, it is something we need to do if we want to extend our lives and live healthier.

Chapter 2: Keto Breakfast Recipes

Since your normal high-carb diet has a lot of variety, your ketogenic diet needs to include the same or you will soon revert to your comfortable eating habits. By tasting a different kind of ketogenic meal every day, you will not get bored, and you will be able to find what works for your palette and what does not.

For breakfast, you need something that will be quick and easy to prepare. It should also be tasty, that way you will start your day in a good mood and with a full stomach. The following recipes offer just that: variety, ease, and taste.

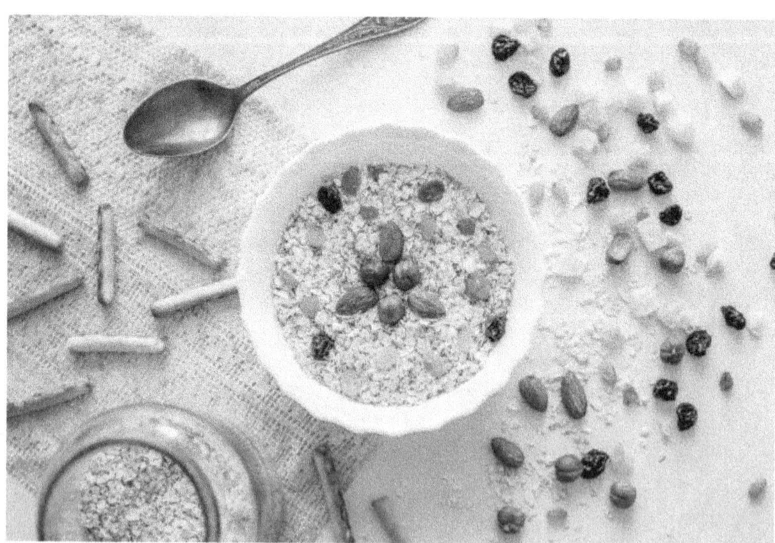

Cheesy Frittata Muffins
Time: 30 minutes

Size: 8 servings

Preparation time: 10 minutes

Cooking time: 20 minutes **Nutritional**

facts/info:

Calories 205

Carbs 1.3 g

Fat 16.1 g

Protein 13.6 g

Ingredients

- 8 large eggs
- 4 oz bacon, pre-cooked and chopped
- 1/2 cup half n' half
- 1 tbsp butter
- 1/2 cup cheddar cheese, shredded
- 1/2 tsp pepper
- 2 tsp dried parsley
- 1/4 tsp salt

Directions

1. Preheat the oven to 375 degrees.

2. Mix the eggs and the half n' half gently in a medium bowl; until it is a little bit scrambled. Make sure that you leave streaks of egg white.

3. Add in the cheese, bacon, and spices. You may also add any additional ingredients to personalize your meal on this step.

4. Grease a muffin tray with butter or a non-stick spray. Try to get a tray that can accommodate 8 frittatas which is what this recipe will yield.

5. Fill each muffin cup to ¾ full.

6. Place the tray into the preheated oven and leave them to bake for 15-18 minutes, or until you see them looking puffy and golden around the edges.

7. Remove from the oven and let sit for about a minute before serving.

Cheesy Scrambled Eggs

Time: 10 minutes

Serving Size:
1 serving **Prep**
Time: 5
minutes **Cook**
Time: 5
minutes
Nutritional
Facts/Info:

Calories 453

Carbs 1.2 g

Fat 43 g

Protein 19 g

Ingredients:

- 2 large eggs
- 1 oz cheddar cheese, shredded
- 2 tbsp butter

Directions:

1. Beat the eggs in a small bowl.

2. Heat the butter in a frying pan (can substitute olive oil).

3. Once the butter has melted, add the 2 eggs.

4. Let the eggs cook slowly, only touching them once or twice during the process.

5. Add cheese on top of the eggs and mix as the cheese melts.

Bulletproof Coffee

Time: 10 minutes

Serving Size:

1 serving

Prep Time: 5 minutes **Cook Time:** 5 minutes

Nutritional Facts/Info:

Calories 273

Carbs 1 g

Fat 30 g

Protein 0 g

Ingredients:

- 1 cup brew coffee
- 1 tbsp coconut oil
- 1 tbsp unsalted butter
- 1 tbsp heavy cream **Directions:**

1. Brew a cup worth of coffee into a large container.
2. Cut off 1 tbsp of butter. Drop the butter into the coffee and watch it melt.
3. Measure out 1 tbsp coconut oil and plunk that into the coffee also.
4. Add 1 tbsp heavy cream to the coffee.
5. Mix well using a hand blender.

Pecan & Coconut & Oatmeal

Time: 10 minutes

Serving Size:
1 serving

Prep Time: 5
minutes **Cook**

Time: 5 minutes

Nutritional Facts/Info:

Calories 312

Carbs 7 g

Fat 25 g

Protein 13.4 g

Ingredients:

- ½ cup coconut or almond milk
- 2 tbsp almond flour
- 2 tsp chia seeds
- 2 tbsp hemp hearts
- 1 tbsp flax meal
- ¼ tsp pure vanilla extract
- ¼ tsp ground cinnamon
- 1 tbsp coconut flakes
- 1 tbsp pecans, toasted and chopped **Directions:**

1. Mix the milk, chia seeds, almond flour, flax meal, hemp hearts, cinnamon, and vanilla in a small pot.

2. Cook everything together over low heat making sure to stir continuously; the mixture should thicken after about 5 minutes.

3. Spoon the mixture into a bowl and top with the pecans and coconut flakes.

Blueberry Almond Pancakes

Time:10 minutes

serving: 10 pancakes **Prep Time:** 5 minutes **Cook Time:** 5 minutes

Nutritional Facts/Info:

Calories 114

Carbs 3.9 g

Fat 10 g

Protein 3.9 g

Ingredients:

- 4 tbsp butter

- ¼ cup almond milk
- 2 large eggs
- ¾ cup almond flour
- ¼ tsp pure vanilla extract
- 1 tbsp flax meal
- 1 packet stevia powder
- 1 tsp baking powder
- ¼ tsp allspice (optional)
- ¼ tsp sea salt
- ¾ cup blueberries, frozen or fresh
- butter, to cook the pancakes **Directions:**

1. Whisk the butter, eggs, almond milk, and vanilla in a small bowl.
2. Add the flour, flax meal, baking powder, stevia, salt, allspice until well blended.
3. Fold in the blueberries.
4. Heat a non-stick skillet over medium heat. You can test if it is ready by dropping small drops of water and they should dance across the surface.
5. Melt a little bit of butter in the pan.
6. Drop scant ¼ cupsful of batter into the skillet, spreading it out into thin circles (they will puff up).
7. Cover the pan with a lid and cook for 1 to 2 minutes, until air bubbles appear on top, and the batter looks a little dry.

8. Flip and cook until golden underneath, 2 minutes more.

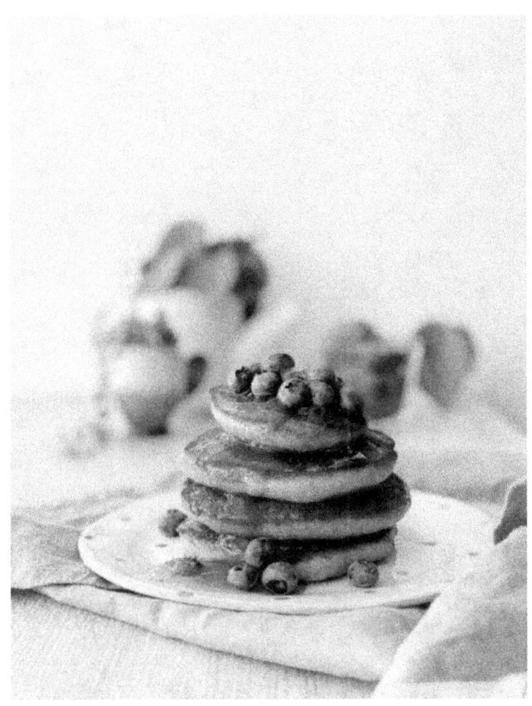

Lemon Poppy Seed Muffins

Time: 30 minutes

Serving Size:

8 muffins

Prep Time: 15 minutes **Cook Time:**

15 minutes **Nutritional Facts/Info:**

Calories 116

Carbs 10 g

Fat 10.7 g

Protein 3.6 g

Ingredients:

- ⅓ cup low-calorie natural sweetener
- ¼ cup coconut flour
- ¼ cup almond flour
- 1 lemon, zested
- 1 tbsp poppy seeds
- ½ tsp salt
- ½ tsp baking powder
- 3 eggs
- ¼ tsp xanthan gum (optional)
- 2 tbsp sour cream

- 3 tbsp butter

- 2 tbsp heavy whipping cream, or more to taste

- ½ tsp vanilla extract

Directions:

1. Preheat the oven to 350 degrees.

2. Line a muffin tin with paper muffin liners or grease a muffin tin with butter.

3. Combine the sweetener, coconut flour, almond flour, poppy seeds, baking powder, lemon zest, salt, and xanthan gum in a medium mixing bowl.

4. Beat eggs until fluffy, 2 minutes on high speed with an electric mixer.

5. Combine the sour cream, butter, and vanilla extract in a mixing bowl. Some sweeteners can be added to the mixture if a sweeter taste is desired.

6. Stir cream in gently until the batter is thick and creamy.

7. Fill each muffin cup to ½ full of batter.

8. Bake in the preheated oven for 15 to 20 minutes, or until the tops are golden.

Almond & Coconut Pancakes

Time: 15 minutes

Serving Size:
8 pancakes

Prep   Time:

10 minutes

Cook Time: 5
minutes

**Nutritional
Facts/Info:**

Calories 383

Carbs 13.4 g

Fat 33.2 g

Protein 15.3 g

Ingredients:

- 1 cup almond flour
- 2 tbsp low-calorie natural sweetener
- ¼ cup coconut flour
- 1 tsp baking powder
- 1 tsp salt
- 6 eggs, at room temperature
- 2 tbsp butter, melted
- ¼ cup heavy whipping cream, at room temperature

- 1 tsp vanilla extract

Directions:

1. Whisk together the almond flour, coconut flour, sweetener, salt, baking powder in a small bowl (can add cinnamon, if desired).
2. Slowly add in the eggs, heavy cream, butter, and vanilla extract until just mixed.
3. Heat oil on a griddle over a medium-high stove.
4. Drop large spoonsful of batter onto the griddle.
5. Cook for 2 to 3 minutes, until browned. Continue process for remaining batter.

Poached Eggs Mytilene

Time: 20 minutes

Serving Size:

1 (2 eggs)

Prep Time:

10   minutes

Cook Time:

10 minutes

Nutritional Facts/Info:

Calories 275

Carbs 6.1 g

Fat 23.6 g

Protein 13.2 g

Ingredients:

- ½ medium lemon, juiced
- 1 tbsp extra-virgin olive oil
- 1 ½ cups water
- 1 ½ tbsp white vinegar
- 2 large eggs
- salt and pepper, to taste **Directions:**

1. Whisk together the lemon juice and oil in a shallow serving bowl.
2. Bring water and vinegar to a slow boil in a shallow pan, then reduce heat to low.
3. Crack 1 egg in a small bowl, being careful not to break the yolk.

4. Slip the egg into the simmering water softly, leaving the bowl slightly above the water's surface. Repeat this process for the remaining egg.

5. Cook for 2 to 3 minutes, or until the whites are solid and the yolks are gently cooked on the outside but still runny on the inside.

6. With a slotted spoon, remove eggs from the water and put in a serving dish.

7. Split the yolks and drizzle with lemon juice mixture, season with salt and pepper.

Chapter 3: Keto Lunch Recipes

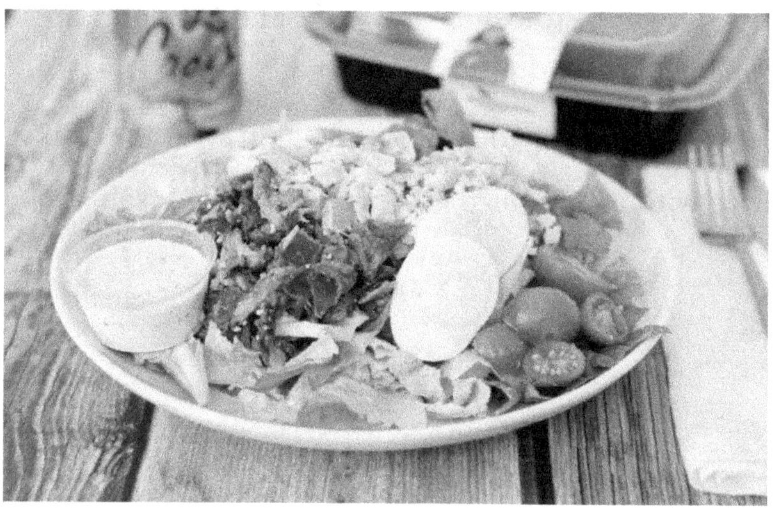

In this section we are still trying to keep things simple and delicious. Variety and efficiency are still the key so that you do not get tired of the same dishes nor lose momentum with the diet.

We often skip lunch because we get too busy to prepare a decent meal. If you think about your eating habits when you are on your high-carb diet, skipping lunch really means snacking on junk. Instead of making a proper meal for lunch, you are more likely to go for anything that is easily accessible. Sometimes it is fruit or nuts, but other times it can be candy or chips.

Cauliflower Mac 'n Cheese
Time: 40 minutes

Serving Size:

4 servings

Prep Time:

15   minutes

Cook Time:

25

minutes

Nutritional

Facts/Info:

Calories 389

Carbs 9.5 g

Fat 35 g

Protein 12 g

Ingredients:

- 1 head cauliflower, cut into florets
- 1 tsp mixed herbs
- 1 tsp salt
- 3 tbsp olive oil
- ½ tsp ground black pepper
- ½ cup heavy whipping cream

- 1 cup cheddar cheese, shredded

- 1 pinch ground nutmeg

- 1 tbsp ghee (clarified butter)

- 3 tbsp parmesan cheese, grated **Directions:**

1. Preheat the oven to 450 degrees.

2. Wrap aluminium foil over a baking sheet.

3. Place cauliflower on the prepared baking sheet.

4. Add salt, pepper, and mixed herbs.

5. Drizzle with olive oil and toss to cover everything.

6. Roast for 10 to 15 minutes in the preheated oven until crisp.

7. Fill an 8-inch baking dish with the mixture.

8. Mix cheddar cheese, heavy cream, ghee, and nutmeg in a saucepan over medium heat; cook until bubbly, around 5 minutes.

9. Pour over cauliflower and toss to blend.

10. Cover with a sprinkling of parmesan cheese and bake again for 10 minutes.

Beef Egg Roll Slaw

Time: 30 minutes

Serving Size:

6 servings

Prep Time:

15   minutes

Cook Time:

15 minutes

Nutritional Facts/Info:

Calories 350

Carbs 12 g

Fat 24g

Protein 20.6g

Ingredients:

- 2 tbsp sesame oil
- ½ cup onion, diced
- 5 green onions, chopped, white and green parts separated
- 3 cloves garlic, minced
- 1 ½ oz ground beef
- 1 tbsp chili-garlic sauce (such as sriracha)
- ½ tsp ground ginger
- 1 (14 oz) package coleslaw mix
- 3 tbsp soy sauce

- 1 tbsp apple cider vinegar

- salt and pepper, to taste

Directions:

1. Heat the oil in a large skillet over a medium-high heat.

2. Add diced onion, green onion whites, and garlic to the pan. After 5 minutes, the onions should be transparent and the garlic fragrant.

3. Combine ground beef, chili-garlic sauce, ginger, salt, and pepper in a large skillet.

4. Cook for about 5 minutes, or until the beef is brown and crumbly.

5. Combine the steak, coleslaw mix, soy sauce, and cider vinegar in a mixing cup.

6. Cook for another 4 minutes, or until the coleslaw is tender.

7. Garnish with the remaining green onions.

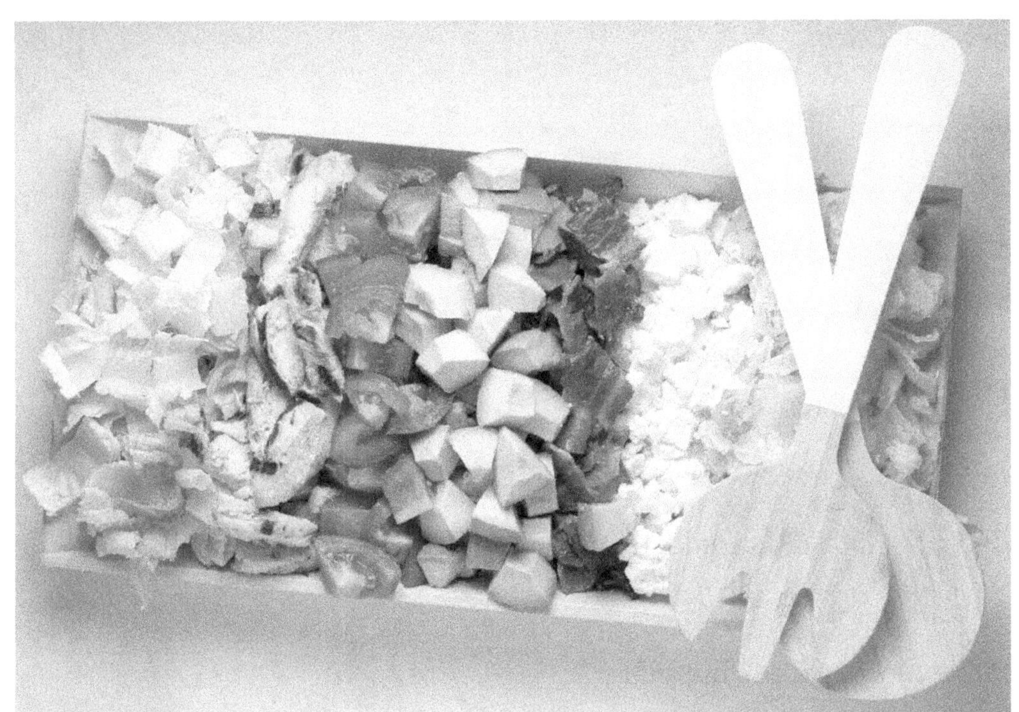

Cobb Salad

Time: 50 minutes

Serving Size:

6 servings

Prep   Time:

20   minutes

Cook Time:

30 minutes

Nutritional

Facts/Info:

Calories 525 Carbs

10.2 g

Fat 39.9 g

Protein 31.7 g

Ingredients:

- 6 slices bacon
- 1 head iceberg lettuce, shredded
- 3 eggs
- 2 tomatoes, seeded and chopped
- 3 cups cooked, chopped chicken breast • 1 avocado, peeled, pitted, and diced
- ¾ cup blue cheese, crumbled
- 1 (8 oz) bottle ranch-style salad dressing
- 3 green onions, chopped **Directions:**

1. Fill a saucepan halfway with cold water and add the eggs.
2. Place the saucepan on a high heat stove and bring to boil.
3. Cover remove from heat, and let eggs sit for 10 to 12 minutes in the hot water.
4. Remove from the hot water and allow to cool before peeling and chopping.

5. Cook the bacon in a deep pan until uniformly browned over medium-high heat.

6. Drain, crumble, and place on a tray.

7. Assemble individual plates of sliced lettuce.

8. On top of the lettuce, equally divide and arrange the chicken, eggs, tomatoes, blue cheese, bacon, avocado, and green onions in a line.

9. Drizzle with your favourite vinaigrette.

Shrimp Scampi with Broccoli Noodles

Time: 30 minutes

Serving Size:
4 servings

Prep Time:
15   minutes

Cook Time:
15 minutes

Nutritional
Facts/Info:

Calories 267 Carbs

12.8 g

Fat 14.2 g

Protein 23.5 g

Ingredients:

- 2 large heads broccoli with long stems
- 2 tbsp olive oil, divided
- 1 pound raw shrimp, peeled and deveined
- 2 cloves garlic, minced
- 2 tbsp lemon juice
- 2 tbsp dry white wine
- 1 tbsp fresh basil, minced
- 2 tbsp butter
- ½ tsp crushed red pepper flakes
- 1 tbsp fresh chives, chopped
- salt and pepper, to taste

Directions:

1. Cut off broccoli florets and store for later use.
2. Break of the asparagus' woody ends; there is a natural breaking point.
3. Shave big knots off the stems using a vegetable peeler; making them as uniform as possible.

4. Spiralize noodles using the smallest setting.

5. Heat 1 tbsp olive oil over medium-high heat in a large skillet.

6. Toss the broccoli noodles with salt and pepper for 3 minutes.

7. Remove the pan from the heat and set it aside.

8. In a separate pan, heat the remaining olive oil and garlic over medium heat for 1 minute.

9. Toss the shrimp into the pan and cook until they are opaque, 3 minutes per side.

10. Place the shrimp in a dish.

11. In the same pan, mix the wine, lemon juice, butter, basil, chives, and red pepper for 3 minutes over medium heat.

12. Toss the shrimp back into the skillet to coat.

13. Place broccoli noodles in serving bowls. Top with the shrimp mixture.

Cucumber Avocado Salad with Bacon

Time: 10 minutes

Serving Size:
2 servings

Prep   Time:
10 minutes

Cook Time: 0
minutes

**Nutritional
Facts/Info:**

Calories 419

Carbs 13 g

Fat 38.3 g

Protein 10.4 g

Ingredients:

- 2 cups fresh baby spinach, chopped
- 1 small avocado, peeled, pitted, and chopped
- ½ English cucumber, sliced thin

- 1 ½ tbsp lemon juice

- 1 ½ tbsp olive oil

- 2 slices cooked bacon, chopped

- salt and pepper, to taste **Directions:**

1. Combine the spinach, cucumber, and avocado in a salad bowl.

2. Combine the olive oil, lemon juice, salt, and pepper in the salad bowl.

3. Top with chopped bacon.

Bacon Cheeseburger Soup

Time: 25 minutes

Serving Size:

4 servings

Prep Time:

10   minutes

Cook Time:

15 minutes

Nutritional

Facts/Info:

Calories 315

Carbs 6 g

Fat 20 g

Protein 27 g

Ingredients:

- 4 slices uncooked bacon
- 1 medium yellow onion, chopped
- 8 oz ground beef (80% lean)
- 3 cups beef broth
- 1 clove garlic, minced
- 2 tsp dijon mustard
- 2 tbsp tomato paste
- 1 cup shredded lettuce
- ½ cup cheddar cheese, shredded

Directions:

1. Fry the bacon until crisp, then drain on paper towels and slice.
2. Reheat the bacon fat before adding the meat.
3. Cook until the beef is golden brown, then remove half of the grease.

4. Cook for 6 minutes after reheating the saucepan and adding the onion and garlic.

5. Add the broth, tomato paste, and mustard.

6. Cover and cook the beef for 15 minutes on medium-low heat.

7. Serve in bowls of shredded lettuce, cheddar cheese, and garnish with bacon.

Ham and Provolone Sandwich

Time: 35 minutes

Serving Size:
1 serving

Prep   Time:
30 minutes

Cook Time: 5
minutes

**Nutritional
Facts/Info:**

Calories 425

Carbs 5 g

Fat 31 g

Protein 31 g

Ingredients:

- 1 large egg, separated
- pinch of salt
- pinch of cream of tartar
- ¼ cup shredded provolone cheese
- 1 oz cream cheese, softened
- 3 oz ham, sliced **Directions:**

1. Preheat the oven to 350 degrees.
2. Beat the egg whites with the cream of tartar and salt until soft peaks form.
3. Combine the cream cheese and egg yolk in a mixing bowl and whisk until smooth and pale yellow.
4. Fold in the egg whites into the cream cheese mixture a little at a time until smooth and well combined.
5. Create two even circles with the batter on the baking dish.
6. Bake for 25 minutes, or until solid and lightly browned.
7. Spread the butter on one side of each bread circle, and place one piece in a preheated skillet over medium heat.
8. Sprinkle with cheese, then finish with sliced ham and the butter-side-up other bread circle.

9. Cook for a minute or two before gently turning it over; ensure cheese melts.

Baked Chicken Nuggets

Time: 30 minutes

Serving Size:

4 servings

Prep Time:

10   minutes

Cook Time:

20 minutes

**Nutritional
Facts/Info:**

Calories 400

Carbs 2 g

Fat 26 g

Protein 43 g

Ingredients:

- ¼ cup almond flour

- ½ tsp paprika

- 1 tsp chili powder

- 2 pounds boneless chicken thighs, cut into 2-inch chunks

- 2 large eggs, whisked well

- salt and pepper, to taste **Directions:**

1. Preheat the oven to 400 degrees.

2. Cover a baking sheet with parchment paper.

3. Combine the almond flour, chili powder, and paprika in a shallow dish.

4. Sprinkle salt and pepper on the chicken before dipping it in the eggs.

5. Dredge chicken chunks in almond mixture and then place on the baking sheet.

6. Cook for 20 minutes, or until golden brown and crisp.

Chapter 4: Keto Dinner Recipes

It is important to prepare the delicious meals for yourself—this will help you stay committed and ensure you know the nutritional value of each meal. Dinner time is often the biggest meal of the day and one that people spend the most time preparing. A nice hack can be to cook more than you need and have leftovers for lunch the next day.

If you have a partner and/or family, dinner is a great mealtime to introduce them to the ketogenic diet, as well. They may resist the reduction in carbohydrates initially, but they just need to give some delicious hearty meals with the carb substitutes a chance. As with any new habit, having an accountability partner can help you stay committed, so getting your partner on the diet with you will benefit you in the long term.

Following are recipes rich in flavour and variety of ingredients to entice even the most reluctant to not only begin the keto diet, but to also want to stick with it.

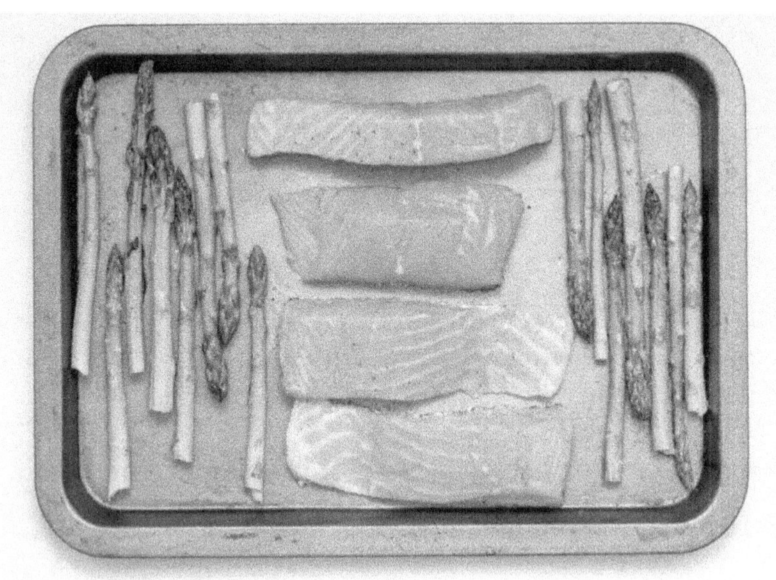

Grilled Pesto Salmon with Asparagus

Time: 20 minutes

Serving Size:

4 servings

Prep Time: 5

minutes **Cook**

Time: 15

minutes

Nutritional

Facts/Info:

Calories 300

Carbs 2.5 g

Fat 17.5 g

Protein 34.5 g

Ingredients:

- 4 (6 oz) boneless salmon fillets
- 1 bunch asparagus, ends trimmed
- 2 tbsp olive oil
- ¼ cup basil pesto
- salt and pepper, to taste **Directions:**

1. Preheat the grill to high and spray the grates with grease.
2. Season the salmon with salt and pepper and then spray it with cooking spray.
3. Grill the salmon for 4 to 5 minutes on either side, or until it is completely cooked.
4. Toss the asparagus with the oil and grill for about 10 minutes, or until tender.
5. Serve the salmon with the pesto on top and asparagus on the side.

Chicken Cordon Bleu with Cauliflower

Time: 55 minutes

Serving Size:

4 servings

Prep Time:

10   minutes

Cook Time:

45 minutes

**Nutritional
Facts/Info:**

Calories 420

Carbs 7 g

Fat 23.5 g

Protein 45 g

Ingredients:

- 4 boneless chicken breast halves (about 12 oz)

- 1 large egg, whisked well

- 4 slices deli ham

- 4 slices swiss cheese

- ¼ cup almond flour • 2 oz pork rinds

- ½ tsp garlic powder

- ¼ cup parmesan cheese, grated

- 2 cups cauliflower florets

- salt and pepper, to taste **Directions:**

1. Preheat the oven to 350 degrees.

2. Cover a baking sheet with aluminium foil.

3. Place the chicken breast halves between parchment paper and pound flat.

4. Arrange the chicken on a serving platter and top with sliced ham and cheese.

5. Wrap the chicken around the filling and then dip in the beaten egg.

6. Pulse the pork rinds, almond flour, parmesan, garlic powder, salt, and pepper into fine crumbs in a food processor.

7. Roll the chicken in the pork rind mixture and then place on the baking sheet.

8. Add the cauliflower to the baking sheet after tossing it in melted butter.

9. Bake for 45 minutes, or until chicken is fully cooked.

Sesame-Crusted Tuna with Green Beans

Time: 20 minutes

Serving Size:
4 servings

Prep   Time:
15 minutes

Cook Time: 5
minutes

**Nutritional
Facts/Info:**

Calories 380

Carbs 8 g

Fat 19 g

Protein 44.5 g

Ingredients:

- ¼ cup white sesame seeds
- ¼ cup black sesame seeds

- 4 (6 oz) ahi tuna steaks

- 1 tbsp olive oil

- 1 tbsp coconut oil

- 2 cups green beans

- salt and pepper, to taste **Directions:**

1. Mix the two forms of sesame seeds in a shallow bowl until it forms a paste.

2. Using salt and pepper, season the tuna.

3. Dredge the tuna using the sesame seed paste.

4. Heat the olive oil in a skillet over high pressure.

5. Add the tuna and cook for 1–2 minutes on one side, then sear on the other.

6. Remove the tuna from the skillet and set it aside to rest while the skillet is reheated with coconut oil.

7. Fry the green beans in the coconut oil for 5 minutes. Serve hot with the sliced tuna.

Lamb Meatballs on Zucchini Noodles

Time: 20 minutes

Serving Size:

4 servings

Prep Time: 5 minutes **Cook Time:** 15 minutes

Nutritional Facts/Info:

Calories 348

Carbs 21.1 g

Fat 4.2 g

Protein 36.1 g

Ingredients:

- 1 lb 2 oz zucchini
- 16 oz pasta sauce
- 1 lb ground lamb
- 2 shallots
- 1 egg yolk
- 1 tsp cinnamon
- 1 tsp cumin
- cayenne pepper, red pepper flakes, to taste
- salt and pepper, to taste **Directions:**

1. Preheat the oven to 450 degrees.

2. Julienne the zucchini using a slicer. Stop only before you get to the seeded part of the zucchini flesh.

3. Combine the remaining ingredients (except the pasta sauce) and shape it into roughly 16 1 oz meatballs.

4. Cook the meatballs for 12 minutes; make sure they are cooked through.

5. Combine the pasta sauce and the baked zucchini noodles in a saucepan and cook for 3 to 4 minutes.

6. Serve alongside meatballs.

Kimchi Pork Lettuce Cups

Time: 20 minutes

Serving Size:

2 servings

Prep Time:

10   minutes

Cook Time:

10 minutes

Nutritional Facts/Info:

Calories 322

Carbs 6.8 g

Fat 24.3 g

Protein 19.7 g

Ingredients:

- 2 tsp extra virgin olive oil
- 1 garlic clove, chopped fine
- 8 oz ground pork
- handful of fresh cilantro, chopped
- ½ cup kimchi, chopped fine
- 1 tsp fish sauce (Red Boat fish sauce has no added sugar)
- 1½ tsp soy sauce
- 1 small head boston lettuce, leaves removed, rinsed, and patted dry
- salt, to taste
- lime wedges, for garnish **Directions:**

1. Heat the oil in a 10-inch skillet over medium-high heat until it shimmers.
2. Sauté the garlic for 1 to 2 minutes, or until it is lightly golden.
3. Add the pork and cut up some big chunks with a fork.
4. Combine the cilantro, kimchi, fish sauce, and soy sauce in a mixing bowl, and season with salt and pepper.
5. Reduce the heat to medium-low and add the cilantro mixture to the pork.

6. Cook, stirring every couple of minutes, for another 7 to 9 minutes, or until the pork is cooked through.

7. Arrange the lettuce leaves on a platter.

8. Cover the lettuce leaves with the fried pork stuffing. Serve with lime wedges.

Thai Turkey Burgers

Time: 15 minutes

Serving Size:
2 servings

Prep Time: 5
minutes **Cook
Time:** 10
minutes
**Nutritional
Facts/Info:**

Calories 451

Carbs 1.8 g

Fat 29 g

Protein 45.5 g

Ingredients:

- 12 oz ground turkey
- 1 garlic clove, finely chopped
- 1 tsp ginger, freshly grated
- handful of fresh cilantro, stems and leaves finely chopped

- 2 tsp red curry paste

- ½ tsp sea salt

- 4 tsp mayonnaise

- ½ tsp dijon mustard

- 2 tsp extra virgin olive oil

- 2 romaine heart leaves or curly kale leaves

- salt and pepper, to taste

Directions:

1. Combine the turkey, garlic, ginger, half of the chopped cilantro, chili paste, and salt in a medium mixing bowl. Mix well.

2. Form the mixture into two 4-inch patties by dividing it into two separate parts.

3. Combine the mayonnaise, dijon, and the remaining cilantro in a shallow bowl.

4. Add salt and pepper to taste.

5. Heat the oil over medium-high heat in a medium skillet.

6. Cook until the burgers are browned on the outside, around 4 or 5 minutes.

7. Cook for another 4 or 5 minutes, or until the other side is browned and cooked through.

8. To eat, wrap each burger in a lettuce leaf.

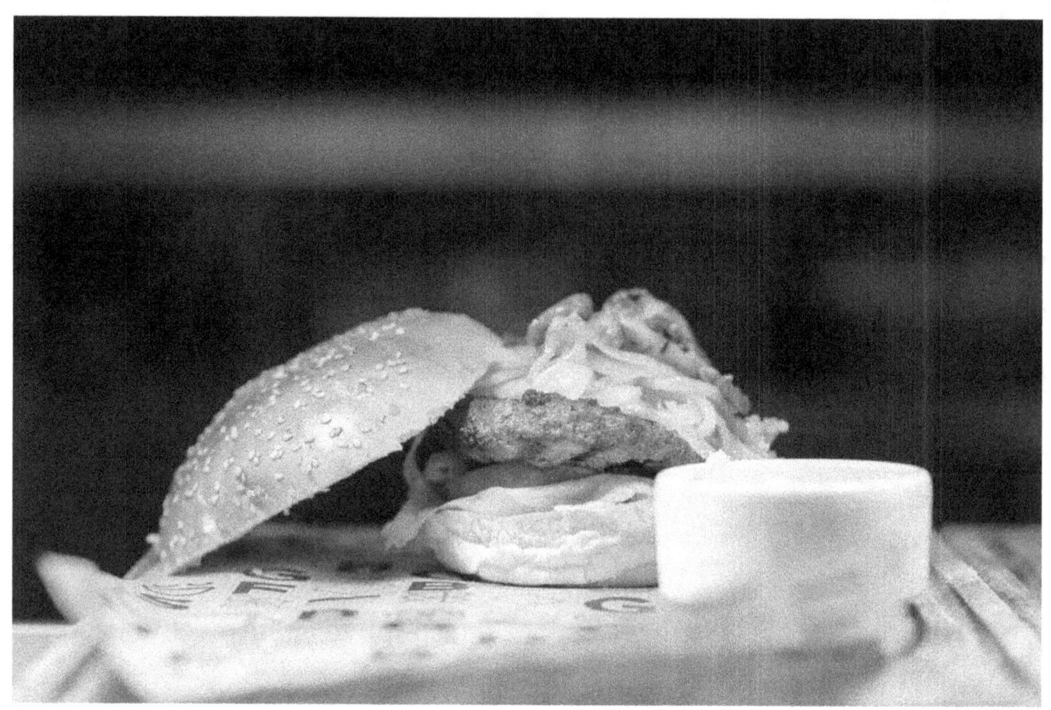

BBQ Flank Steak & Cabbage Slaw

Time: 20 minutes

Serving Size:

2 servings

Prep Time: 5 minutes **Cook Time:** 15 minutes

Nutritional Facts/Info:

Calories 392

Carbs 3 g

Fat 25 g

Protein 37 g

Ingredients:

- ¼ cup ketchup (a no-sugar-added variety, such as Primal Kitchen)
- 2 tbsp butter, melted
- 1 tsp dijon mustard
- ½ tsp onion powder
- ½ tsp worcestershire sauce
- ½ tsp freshly ground black pepper
- 1½ lb flank steak
- ¼ cup mayonnaise
- 1 tbsp apple cider vinegar

- ¼ tsp celery seed

- 2 cups cabbage, shredded

- salt and pepper, to taste **Directions:**

1. Set the broiler to high and place a rack under the broiler pan.

2. Whisk together the ketchup, butter, vinegar, onion powder, worcestershire sauce, and black pepper in a shallow bowl to combine.

3. On a rimmed sheet plate, position the steak.

4. Apply the sauce to the entire surface, including the top and bottom.

5. Cook for 5 to 7 minutes, or until the surface is well browned.

6. Cook for another 5 to 7 minutes, or until target readiness is reached.

7. Allow 5 minutes for the meat to rest.

8. Prepare the slaw, in the meantime, by whisking together the mayonnaise, vinegar, and celery seed in a shallow bowl.

9. Sprinkle some salt and pepper to taste.

10. Stir in the cabbage until it is thoroughly combined, refrigerate until ready to use.
    This can be made up to a day ahead of time.

11. Slice the steak, cutting against the grain, and serve with the slaw.

Beef Bolognese

Time: 3 hours 30 minutes

Serving Size:

4 servings

Prep   Time:

30 minutes

Cook Time: 3
hours

**Nutritional
Facts/Info:**

Calories 532

Carbs 8.4 g

Fat 36.2 g

Protein 42.6 g

Ingredients:

- 4 slices thick-cut bacon, chopped
- 1½ lb ground beef
- ¾ cup heavy cream
- 1 can (28 oz) tomato purée
- zoodles, ready to serve
- grated parmesan cheese, for garnish **Directions:**

1. In a cold deep skillet, cook the bacon over medium-high heat.

2. Cook, turning once, until crisp all over.

3. Using a slotted spoon, transfer to a plate.

4. In a pan, crumble the meat.

5. Cook, stirring regularly, for 5 to 7 minutes, or until well browned.

6. Reduce the heat to a low setting. Add the milk and mix well.

7. Cook, stirring regularly, for about 10 minutes, or until the milk has almost evaporated but the meat is not dry.

8. Scrape up some browned pieces from the bottom of the plate before adding the tomato purée.

9. Bring to a boil then reduce the heat to a low setting.

10. Cook for 2 to 3 hours, stirring occasionally.

11. Add a few tbsp of water, as needed, to prevent the sauce from sticking to the pan.

12. About 30 minutes before the sauce is ready, begin preparing the zoodles.

13. Serve the Bolognese over the zoodles.

Conclusion

The ketogenic diet needs commitment, but it is a commitment that you will reap great benefits from. Weight loss is the primary reason most people turn to the ketogenic diet as with its low carb composition you are guaranteed to shed the pounds quickly. This is due to the key process behind the diet, ketogenesis, which ensures that fat reserves instead of glucose is used for energy. Even though the initial weight loss is why many begin the keto diet, it is for the long-term health benefits that people stick with it.

To aid in long term commitment, it is helpful to ease into the diet and then later transition into a full ketogenic diet. As well, understanding what ketosis is and how to stay under a ketogenic state for longer will benefit the overall effectiveness. It can take time to get used to the process depending on your eating habits prior to starting, and some people's bodies can go into a bit of shock in the beginning as they learn to adjust to the body using ketones for energy. However, it does become easier when you understand the mechanisms of ketosis and stick strictly to the appropriate foods.

To ensure that maximum benefits are gained, and minimum adverse effects are felt, it is critical to manage the ketogenic diet correctly from the start. A suggestion to help with this management would be to plan out a full week of meals, gather all the needed ingredients, remove restricted foods from the home, and weight/measure yourself. Obviously, things can happen which can cause disruptions, but if you do fall off the diet, try to identify what may have gone wrong, adjust, and then try again.

Many things in life that are good for us are often difficult to start and even more difficult to sustain. Diets are a well-known example of this, as they are known to be good for our health but very few people commit to them long-term. An added layer to this lack of commitment is that we have also become addicted to our high calorie convenient meals. All diets need patience and commitment, and the ketogenic diet is no different.

Any time we commit to a significant change in our habits it is important to be careful. Even though the ketogenic diet has been proven beneficial for weight loss and an overall healthy lifestyle, individuals have different underlying factors that they are living with. If you are unsure at all about starting any diet, you want to consult your doctor. As well, if you start the diet and begin to feel any adverse effects, consult your doctor before continuing. Now is the time to make a decision that will change your life for the better; to decide to be a good steward of your body—you will not regret it. The benefits are immense and there is much more to gain than to lose.

References

15 Keto Breakfast Ideas for Going Low-Carb. (n.d.). Allrecipes. Retrieved March 1,
2021, from https://www.allrecipes.com/gallery/keto-breakfast-ideas/

Gunnars, K. (2018, November 20). *10 health benefits of low-carb and ketogenic diets.* Healthline. https://www.healthline.com/nutrition/10-benefits-oflow-carbketogenic-diets

McDonald, L. (1998). *The ketogenic diet: a complete guide for the dieter and practitioner*. Lyle McDonald.

Olsen, N. (2019, March 29). *Ketogenic diet for type 2 diabetes: Side effects, benefits, and alter*. www.medicalnewstoday.com. https://www.medicalnewstoday.com/articles/317431#the-ketogenicdiet-anddiabetes

Spritzler, F. (2020, October 16). *Foods to eat on a ketogenic diet*. Healthline. https://www.healthline.com/nutrition/ketogenic-dietfoods#TOC_TITLE_HDR_2

All images have been sourced from https://unsplash.com/

www.ingramcontent.com/pod-product-compliance
Lightning Source LLC
Chambersburg PA
CBHW080034260726
48658CB00007B/2609